AF207899

# YOU WANT ME TO... WHAT?

## THE UPS AND DOWNS, THE INS AND OUTS:

## THE A-Zs OF NURSING AT ITS BEST

ANTOINETTE LAMBERT, AGPCNP-BC

ISBN 979-8-35091-752-9

eBook ISBN 979-8-35091-753-6

# ACKNOWLEDGEMENTS

Lots of love to my husband Jon who has always encouraged me to step out of my comfort zone.

Love and thanks to my son Will who, by virtue of always striving to reach higher goals, has been a tremendous source of encouragement and inspiration for me.

A big fat thank you to Claudia Alonzo, MA, for her editing.

You Want Me to … What?

# PRIVACY STATEMENT

In order to protect the privacy of the patients and their families, some details have been changed.

Antoinette Lambert, AGPCNP-BC

# *A* IS FOR ANUS. · *A* IS FOR ALLERGY, ANASTOMOSIS, ANEURYSM, AND ACNE.

# *A* IS ALSO FOR AGATHA.

Agatha was a 63-year-old woman who lived with her husband, Adam. They had two children-one son, one daughter – who lived out of town. Agatha, like most aging women and mothers, did not want to worry her children. She did not tell her children that it was getting harder to walk up the steps to the only bathroom in their old home. She did not tell them she wore thick pads in her underwear, so that when she had to urinate, she would just stand and pee. Agatha would then walk on her arthritic knees, rocking side to side as she walked on her bad hip, to her bedroom. There, she would sit until she was able to catch her breath. Her morbid obesity was a topic Agatha did not like to discuss with anyone – not Adam, not her children, not even her doctor. Her morbid obesity was also something she could not ignore, as it made every step and every activity a monumental task that stole her energy and her breath. Once she was able to breathe normally, she would change her pad. She wrapped the soiled pads as best as she could, and would throw them in the trash, where they sat until Adam took out the garbage.

Agatha had been admitted to the hospital after she had fevers and a foul odor coming from her groin area for three or four days. She didn't want to go, but Adam told her he couldn't take the odor any longer. It was when the ER nurses were helping her get undressed that they noted a wound about four inches in diameter in her left groin. The drainage was almost a neon green, with a distinctly sweet smell. Agatha had a pseudomonas aeruginosa infection.

I met Agatha on my weekend rotation. As I received the report, my mind began to picture this obese woman who was as wide as she was tall, unkempt, demanding – someone who would complain that the kitchen brought her three sugars for her oatmeal, when she ordered four! I could feel this heaviness spread across my chest. I knew this feeling. It was *Goddammit, why me?*, accompanied by the oh-so-common sigh. Every nurse knows this feeling (if you say you don't – you're lying).

When I entered the room, I had to do a double-take. Sitting on the edge of the bed was a woman, who was, in fact, nearly as wide as she was tall. Agatha's graying hair had been recently washed, and was stiff from the spray she used to keep every strand in place. Her pudgy fingers were capped with beautifully manicured and painted nails, and a gold ring adorned every finger. Toes were done in the same deep red. Lashes were lengthened with her Maybelline mascara, and lips were a subtle rose from her Burt's Bees lip moisturizer.

As we got to know each other, Agatha related to me the story of her first husband's death. He worked hard as an assembly worker in a shop. He liked to drink as hard as he worked.

One winter night, as Agatha's husband was leaving a bar with some friends, he didn't notice a patch of ice that had formed on the sidewalk, due to snow melting off the bar's roof and freezing when it hit the cold ground. Her husband slipped and fell, hitting his head.

His friends took him home, thinking he just needed to sleep off his alcohol. What they didn't know is that he suffered a brain bleed, which grew larger as he at first slept, and then slipped into unconsciousness and died. This left Agatha with two children under the age of eight to raise on her own. She had never worked, as her husband had been making enough money to support the family.

Needing to get to work as quickly as she could, Agatha took a cleaning job. She cleaned offices and homes. Being a stickler, she would often clean baseboards and floors on her hands and knees. She didn't think to wear knee pads. After her children would go to bed, she would eat to try to squash her grief, her sadness, and her fear.

As Agatha began to cry as she told me this, a bit of her mascara ran down her cheek, mixed with her tears. I began to feel a different sort of feeling in my chest. This new feeling was a sense of admiration, admiration for a woman who did what she could to raise her children, a woman who didn't depend on the government or handouts. I admired this woman who could hardly walk because of her arthritic knees and still took pride in her appearance.

Of course, in trying to gather more information on why she was in the hospital, I asked her, "Agatha, what happened to cause the wound you have?" Agatha raised her right arm, hand at shoulder height, and bobbed her hand up and down in a motion I can only compare to a man simulating masturbating – with a three foot long penis. Imagine the look on my face! I'm not sure how long my stared lasted. It may have been a few seconds, but it seemed like minutes before Agatha stated, "Curtain rod." "Excuse me?" I pressed. "I can't reach, so when I get an itch, I scratch with a curtain rod," she explained. Well…of course. How silly of me. Doesn't everyone?

Agatha was treated with antibiotics, her wound managed by the wound clinic. Our social worker was able to set her up with home services, which included a bath aid. She never returned to our hospital with another wound.

Remember the scene from the Carol Burnett show, where she walks down the stairs with a curtain rod across her shoulders, wearing the curtains in place of an elegant dress? Since I met Agatha, I've never been able to look at window dressing the same.

$\mathscr{B}$ **IS FOR BUTTOCKS.** $\mathscr{B}$ **IS FOR BRAIN, BARIUM, BOTOX, AND BARORECEPTOR.**

$\mathscr{B}$ **IS ALSO FOR BEN.**

Ben was a 17-year-old male, who came to the hospital from a boys home. He was a chubby, likable, naïve kid. He enjoyed playing video games with his friends, eating hamburgers, and he enjoyed skate-boarding even though he wasn't very good at it. Ben also liked being accepted.

According to records, his father was not a very kind and loving man. Ben was the youngest of three siblings, having an older brother and sister. While his mother was pregnant with him, his parents' marriage became rocky. His father drank too much. When he did, Ben became his target. Ben could never do anything right. He would be made to sit at the family dinner table and, if he was allowed to eat at all, eat bologna, while the rest of the family ate steak, pizza, and any other food a young child would love to have. Whippings with a belt were common.

To escape the fear and sadness at home, Ben would hang out with friends in the woods near his home. There he learned to climb the highest, smallest limbs on trees. He learned how to shoot at squirrels with a slingshot. The woods are also where Ben learned how to smoke weed, and handle a gun.

Ben's attitude began to change. He became mouthier at home and would talk back to his parents. When his father threatened to beat him with a belt, instead of his insides shaking like they used to, he would dare his father to try. Even though he did not have a gun, Ben would tell his father he would get a gun and shoot him while he slept, if he laid hands on him. His parents were at a loss as to how to manage this behavior.

This took care of itself one afternoon when Ben was with some friends at a convenient store. According to Ben, one of the boys stole some items, including a pack of cigarettes, and a mini bottle of alcohol. The clerk saw him, and started to chase the boys. One friend was behind him, and as he was pushing Ben to hurry and get out of the store, he slipped the bottle of alcohol into Ben's pocket. The boys were caught, and the police were called. Reaching their last straw, his parents sent him to a boys home.

I began to hear rumors that the ER was seeing a rash of boys from this home. One young man, in desperation to get out of the home, swallowed dishwasher soap. What the other boys may not have known is that this caused severe burns in his mouth and esophagus, necessitating a transfer to a university setting for a higher level of care. Other boys swallowed things like pennies.

When I met Ben, I was working in endoscopy. I was told we were going to do an EGD (place a camera through his mouth into his stomach) to retrieve a foreign object.

Ben had already been to Xray. We were told the object was close to the pyloric sphincter (the opening at the bottom of the stomach that lets food pass into the intestine).

It turns out, Ben had swallowed a screw. We performed our procedure, looking into the first part of the intestine, and were unable to find the screw. It had already passed beyond the reaches of our scope.

Once Ben was awake and the sedation had worn off, he asked me if we had removed the screw. I had to tell him we were unable to reach it. The doctors would continue to watch him and take X-rays to watch the progression of the screw. He was silent for a minute, and then said, "I sure hope I swallowed it upside down."

Me too, buddy. Me too.

# *C* IS FOR COLON. *C* IS FOR CATATONIA, COCCYX, CRANIUM, AND CARDIOPULMONARY RESUSCITATION.

# *C* IS ALSO FOR CARL.

Carl was a single, 54-year-old male who was in the ICU due to sepsis. He had begun running fevers at home, where his symptoms progressed to nausea, abdominal pain, and weakness. When he had trouble standing because he was so weak, 911 was called.

The ER did the typical workup: blood work, urine sample, chest X Ray, and an abdominal CT (cat scan) to try to locate the source of his abdominal pain. Carl was found to have several abscesses in his abdomen. He was showing signs of sepsis – decreasing blood pressure and increased effort in breathing, so he was admitted to the ICU.

Antibiotics were started after a large IV line was placed in the right side of Carl's neck. Fluids were infused to help maintain his blood pressure. A catheter was inserted into his bladder, for every drop of urine to be measured. Carl also had a catheter placed in an artery in his arm so accurate blood pressure measurements could be taken.

While calling the emergency numbers in his chart, the secretary spoke to Carl's sister Wendy. Wendy stated that Carl had been living with his mother, Mary. Mary was 83, and had been in a nursing home for two years due to dementia and other health problems. Carl, who had never left home for reasons Wendy did not share, had been having a difficult time adjusting to living without his mother. He could go days without bathing. He may only eat once a day.

Carl had been in our ICU for almost three weeks when I left for a weeklong vacation. He had been placed on medication to help keep his blood pressure up. A tube had been placed in his rectum so the diarrhea he was having did not ulcerate his skin. Nutrition was provided by a small tube that ran through his nose into his stomach. BiPAP was used on and off to help his work of breathing and keep his oxygen level up. When he wasn't responding well to the antibiotics, Carl was taken to surgery and had a drain placed in each of his abscesses. The drains gave the illusion he had an octopus coming from his abdomen.

When I returned from vacation, Carl was not in his usual room. I was told he dropped his blood pressure again, but with all the interventions tried, Carl still died. The staff had been in contact with Wendy through all this. Wendy told the staff her mother had also died – the same day Carl passed away – less than ninety minutes before Carl. Cue the Outer Limits music.

I cannot see the wind, but I see its effects. I believe there is power out there which cannot be seen but has an effect on each one of us in some fashion. All sorts of theories started circulating in our ICU. Perhaps Carl knew, in some way, his mother died, and he decided he was going to go be with her. After all, he didn't like being without her. The love a mother has for her children is like no other. Maybe Mary died, and her soul worked its way to our ICU, and she came to take Carl with her.

As the mother of a son, my heart votes for the latter.

# $\mathscr{D}$ IS FOR DEBRIDEMENT. $\mathscr{D}$ IS FOR DUODENUM, DEXTROSE, DEFIBRILLATOR, AND DIARRHEA.

# $\mathscr{D}$ IS ALSO FOR DIANE.

Diane was a 56-year-old female who came in for her colonoscopy. She had not been having any symptoms – no bloating, no pain, no blood in her stools. What she did have was a family history of colon cancer. It stole her mother away at the young age of 68. Diane did not know until too late that her mother was ill. Mom had been losing some weight, but Diane just assumed it was because she was on one of her 'fad diets,' as Diane called them. When her mother had episodes of unexpected confusion, Diane insisted her mother go to the ER. A head CT revealed a brain lesion, appearing "consistent with metastasis." An abdominal CT was then done, which showed a mass in the sigmoid colon, and also the liver. Diane was in shock. Then she was pissed. Her mother told her she had been having some symptoms – blood in her stools, some belly pain – but she was afraid to get checked. She was afraid to find out she might have cancer. Besides, Diane's mother told her, no one is putting anything "up there."

Diane had done her prep the day before, drinking the liquid that would cause her to make friends with her favorite toilet several times throughout the day. As part of the usual procedure preparation, we asked Diane when she last ate anything solid, or drank any liquid. She had followed all of the directions perfectly. She did not want to have to do this twice! We started an IV, and began slowly infusing normal saline. Eventually we would use her IV site to give her the sleepy medications for the procedure, her conscious sedation.

The medications we used at the time were Versed and Demerol. Versed was used for sedation, to give a patient that "twilight sleep," and for its amnesic benefits. Demerol was to help with any pain that might be encountered, and to aid sedation. Most people don't want to remember their colonoscopy. The two medications worked well together and also made people say some crazy things. Getting a six-foot long scope through a colon was not as easy as the textbooks would lead you to believe. There were twists and turns presenting challenges. The air used to insufflate (open up) the colon could cause pain and cramping.

To start the procedure, Diane was lying on her left side. There was a monitor in front of her. This is where we would visualize Diane's deep, dark…. colon. The doctor and I were standing behind her, as I began slowly administering her sedation. The more difficult part of the procedure is getting the colonoscope around the large intestine, to the point where it joins the small intestine. Once there, we snap a photo, and the doctor then begins the task of slowly withdrawing the scope. Withdrawing the scope is the easier portion of the procedure, but also the most important. We don't want to miss anything that could be cancerous, or potentially morph into cancer in the future. Once we make it to the end of the large intestine, as long as the patient is comfortable, we do not give any more sedation, and we let the patient begin to wake up.

As Diane began to wake up, still a bit foggy from her medication, she could feel the colonoscope in her rectum. Occasionally as the doctor had to reposition the scope, his gloved hand would bump her buttocks. Suddenly, Diane was flapping her hand towards her bottom, saying, "Sam! Stop it. Stop it, Sam." My eyes grew as big as frisbees. I whipped my head to look at the doctor, and he was looking at me. "Who's Sam?" he asked. "I don't know, and I don't want to know," I replied. "Just keep going and get the heck outta there!"

We completed the procedure without any complications. As we wheeled Diane to her recovery room, she asked, "Did I say anything stupid?" "Uh….ummm…nope. You were fine," was all I could think to say. As we pushed her cart into her room, I was startled to see a gentleman sitting in a chair in the corner. "You must be Sam?" I greeted him. "Yes. I'm Diane's husband," he answered. I handed Diane over to her very capable recovery nurse, and high-tailed it back to the endoscopy unit, trying not to giggle out loud.

Oh. You'll be happy to know, Diane had no signs of cancer.

# $\mathscr{E}$ IS FOR ESOPHAGUS. $\mathscr{E}$ IS FOR ENTEROCOCCUS, ERYTHROMYCIN, EVACUATION, AND EARWAX.

# $\mathscr{E}$ IS ALSO FOR EDNA.

Edna was a 92-year-old woman I met my first month of being an RN – a "real nurse". I was working the 11pm-7am shift on a medical/surgical unit that specialized in renal conditions (disorders of the kidneys). I don't even remember why Edna was admitted to the hospital, but I sure remember my encounter with her.

One thing I prided myself on back then was my ability to make my patients comfortable. We were taught in school not to just check vital signs and perform physical assessments. We also got them their water for the night, fluffed their pillows, and rubbed their backs.

Edna was a frail, thin woman with white curly hair, and blue veins that coursed through her arms. I could count her ribs, and see her prominent sacrum through her paper-thin skin. She did not have an ounce of fat on her. I knew she was a high risk for skin breakdown and wounds, so I wanted to be extra careful, turning her every two hours and cushioning her body well. As I introduced myself to Edna, she made eye contact but did not answer any of my questions. Given the shape her body was in, I had guessed it was consuming all her energy just to breathe. Talking was too much of an effort.

Explanations were given: *Edna, I'm going to check your blood pressure. OK, Edna, I'm going to listen to your heart and lungs. Now, Edna, I'm going to turn you on your left side.* Pillows were placed under her head to support her neck, and between her knees to keep her bony joints from pressing against each other. Before placing two pillows behind her to keep her from rolling backwards, lotion was warmed between my hands, and gently rubbed on to her back. The covers were pulled up to her shoulders, the call light strategically placed within reach. Bedside table in reach: check! I made eye contact with Edna, and asked her if there was anything else I could do for her before I shut her light off. She wrestled her right arm out from under the covers, and began to reach her arm up to me. Thinking she may want to tell me something, I leaned over, and turned my left ear to her. That is when she put her hand on my neck, and kissed my left cheek. I looked at her, and we both smiled.

"Good night, Edna. Sleep well. I'll see you in a couple of hours."

When I went back two hours later to turn her, Edna was dead.

That was in 1987. Some things you just never forget. When I taught, I shared with my students this story. I let them know how I shiver inside sometimes, thinking of how I would feel had my encounter with Edna been rushed, uncaring, task oriented instead of care oriented. I would feel sick to this day knowing Edna's last interaction with someone – me – made her feel as if she were an inconvenience, rather than a human being deserving of compassion and kindness.

I told my students, "Never forget. Never."

# *F* IS FOR FACELIFT. *F* IS FOR FACTOR V, FALLOPIAN TUBE, FANCONI'S SYNDROME, AND FATTY LIVER.

# *F* IS ALSO FOR FRANK.

Frank was a 68-year-old man I met while working on a medical/surgical unit. Frank was a bubbly talker. He had retired from working in a manufacturing facility. It was hard, physical work and Frank was looking forward to having a relaxing retirement. He enjoyed playing cards with his buddies, fishing with his grandkids, traveling, and sex. Frank wanted to continue to have lots of sex with his wife ( I never met her – so I'm not sure how she felt about this). He certainly was not shy about the subject.

Unfortunately, Frank was not able to perform as well as he liked. Frank, like so many other men, had erectile dysfunction. He wasn't always able to obtain an erection, and there were times when he did, it was too soft for penetration. According to Frank, he and his wife had gone through all the emotions a couple can experience. She didn't feel attractive anymore; she thought Frank was having an affair. Frank began to feel "less of a man", because he could no longer satisfy his wife. Their love, however, was strong enough to help them survive this emotional turmoil, and together they began to explore solutions.

He started with labs and a physical exam, which all checked out normally. Frank's doctor then prescribed a series of medications to help him achieve an erection. Several worked at first, but over time became less effective. Others worked also, but would make him feel tired and dizzy throughout the day. He even received a prescription for a medication he would have to inject into his penis. It sounded like a good idea so he took the medication and the syringes home. When it came time to actually give himself the injection, Frank stated his hands started to shake and he began to sweat, almost passing out. This option was no longer a consideration.

The next option he explored was a penile prosthesis. This is a device that is placed surgically. There are two….OK. Before I go on, any men reading this may want to sit down…or leave the room. Good? OK…where was I? Oh, yes. The penis. There are two cylinders which are placed on either side of the penis. These cylinders are connected to a reservoir. The fluid filled reservoir is placed in the lower abdomen, and a small pump is implanted in the scrotum. In order to achieve an erection, the man presses on the pump. This allows fluid from the reservoir to flow into the two cylinders, causing an erect penis. After intercourse, the pump is again pressed, and the fluid flows backwards from the cylinders, into the reservoir. Voila!

As with any surgery, there are risks; there can be complications with the prosthesis. And wouldn't you know, Frank was in our hospital because he experienced a complication. After having the penile prosthesis for just over a year, the pump had begun to erode through his scrotal sac.

Now, I don't have male parts down there, but as Frank was telling me this, I could feel all the muscles in my pelvis start to cramp. Then, all of a sudden I heard him say, "Wanna see?" What happened next seemed to occur in slow motion.

As I raised my right arm to say, "No. That's ok!" Frank's right hand had grabbed his covers, and flung them to the side.

There, in all their glory for me to see, were Frank's penis and scrotum. I'm admittedly not a rocket scientist, but it was awfully hard not to notice the hole in Frank's scrotum. All the while, he was smiling, as if he just won some type of award. I asked if he had pain. "Nope. None." I didn't notice any odor either, thank God. Now this odd occurrence was turning into a *That's so cool!* moment. As I looked closer, performing my assessment (with gloved hands), Frank said, "Watch this." He reached towards his scrotum and squeezed the pump, which appeared as this small, opaque device. I had visions of the Terminator – human skin over this robotic shell. Let's just say, the device still worked.

The decision was made to remove the device, treat Frank with antibiotics and replace the prosthesis in the future. More modern approaches include removing the entire device, washing out the area and replacing the implant, all in one surgery.

Frank made a successful recovery. As far as I am aware, he – and maybe his wife – is living happily ever after.

# ***G*** IS FOR GASTROCNEMIUS. ***G*** IS FOR GAMMA KNIFE, GANGRENE, GASTROPARESIS, AND GYNECOMASTIA.

# ***G*** IS ALSO FOR GEORGE.

George was a 37-year-old male, who had a job working as a welder. He had a beat up pickup, and a one hundred pound mutt named Dog. George had a scar on his left cheek from an old fight, he said. He had hazel eyes, a small space between his front teeth, and two little girls under the age of eight. George also had a drinking problem.

Drinking in his twenties was more binge drinking, he told me. George would party on the weekends with buddies and drink so much he might vomit where he was standing, and drink some more. He passed out on more than one occasion – more than he could count on both hands. Somehow, the binge drinking turned into a couple of beers at home every night after work. When he started to wake up shaky, not feeling well, he realized a beer took the edge off. Knowing he couldn't go to work "smelling like booze", George started putting vodka in his juice at breakfast, and into his work thermos.

Next thing he knew, his belly was getting bigger. George thought he was just putting on weight from the drinking. He didn't get worried until he started getting odd bruises, and his gums would bleed when he brushed his teeth. A thorough workup by his doctor revealed George had liver cirrhosis. The alcohol was taking a toll on his bone marrow; his red blood cell count and platelet counts were low. He had been admitted in the past for blood and platelet infusions. When he was hospitalized, George's parents would keep his girls.

On this particular night, I was paged on my beeper – yup, my beeper. I was told we had a GI bleed, and we were going to scope a patient. The patient happened to be George. It was almost 2 am when we met each other. George told me he had not been feeling well, and that when he vomited blood at home, he took his girls to his parents, telling the girls he would see them in the morning.

We prepped George for the procedure – IV started, fluid infusing, heart monitor attached, numbing spray sprayed to the back of his throat, mouth block in place (to keep his teeth apart, preventing him from biting down on the scope), and sedation meds given.

The medication to numb the throat, cetacaine spray, is pretty powerful. Some people, however, have a sensitive gag reflex. George was one of them. As the physician inserted the scope, George began to gag. Many times, I could talk to the patients and calm them. Not George. He continued to gag, and would reach his hands up towards his face in an attempt to remove whatever his brain perceived as something that certainly should not be in his throat. The physician tried to look into George's esophagus and stomach, yelling at me and the other nurse to hold George still. We fought to hold his hands down and we administered him more sedation. He then gagged hard enough to now start bleeding. George apparently caused enough pressure in his esophagus that he burst an esophageal varice (a varicose vein in the esophagus). Now the crap had hit the fan. We opened his fluid wide up and paged the nursing supervisor to come help us STAT. We told her we would need packed cells immediately to start a blood transfusion… in the endoscopy unit, at 2:45 am.

As we were dealing with all of this, for a moment, our attention was drawn away from the heart monitor. As I put my attention back on his vital signs, George's heart rate was now 30. George was no longer fighting us. 25……19…….shit, shit, shit!

George had no palpable pulse. The physician quickly pulled the scope out of George's stomach as the other nurse and I placed him on his back. We started CPR, but with every compression, there was a small amount of blood that erupted from George's mouth. We were trying to protect his airway, and protect ourselves from the spray of his blood. The code team arrived, and after fifteen minutes we were unable to get his heart restarted. In a room that looked like a brutal murder took place, George was dead.

Two little girls who thought they would wake up and see their father no longer had a father. A mother and father who thought they would have lunch with their son that day were no longer ever going to have another meal with him. Alcohol stole George's life. It put a scar on his girls' childhood. It robbed his parents of future opportunities to tell him they love him (and it ruined a favorite pair of my nursing shoes!).

Please, please, please – if you have a drug or alcohol problem, seek help. Don't think it will go away. Don't think you can handle it alone. Don't think it's not that big a deal. For George's family, it proved to be a horrendous deal.

$\mathscr{H}$ **IS FOR HEMORRHOID.** $\mathscr{H}$ **IS FOR HEMIARTHROPLASTY, HEMANGIOMA, HEMOGLOBIN, AND HEMISPHERE.**

$\mathscr{H}$ **IS ALSO FOR HELEN.**

Helen was a 76-year-old woman with lots to do. She didn't have time for health problems. She wanted to get fixed so she could get back to her house and her garden and her lunch dates.

In her childhood, Helen's mother was a stay-at-home mom, who did the laundry, cleaned, and cooked. According to Helen, "No one beat my mama's cooking!" Everything was cooked in butter or lard. Fried chicken and mashed potatoes dripping with butter were staples. Pies were homemade; crusts made with lard. Even bacon was fried in butter in Helen's house!

Though she was never a large woman, Helen realized she needed to change her diet, when she was around 53. She had developed abdominal pain, which she attributed to constipation. When everything she ate began to bring on pain and make her nauseated, Helen went to her doctor. A workup showed she had gallstone and she had her gallbladder removed. At first, she didn't change her diet. She kept experiencing pain, nausea, and "foul stools". Then she thought, *Maybe I should follow the doctor's advice.* Helen began to eat a cleaner diet of less fat and more fruits and vegetables. Her pain and stinky poop improved! But by then, the damage was already done.

Also in her 70s, Helen began to have random episodes of getting sweaty, nauseated, and dizzy. She drank more water, and took rest breaks between baking pies and doing her laundry. Her symptoms eased, but only for a short while. One Sunday, while in church, the up and down and sitting and kneeling motions began to cause a feeling in her chest that she never had before. It began as pressure, but then evolved into a stabbing pain in her upper back. She was "a bit" lightheaded, but she didn't want to disrupt the service. It was after the preacher said his final prayer that Helen told her friends she needed to go to the hospital. Not wanting an expensive ambulance bill, she had her friends drive her to the hospital.

Helen was in the midst of a heart attack, a STEMI, to be exact. She was given nitroglycerine under her tongue, which relieved some of her pain. Oxygen was placed in her nose via a plastic tubing some patients have told me smells like new tires. Cardiology was called, and the on-call team came in to take Helen to the cardiac cath lab. This is where she would be sedated, the physician would insert a catheter in her groin, thread it up to her heart, and inject dye so the physician could visualize the arteries in her heart. If any of Helen's arteries were determined to be occluded with plaque, the doctor had a few options. One would be to place a stent in the artery to help keep it open. Another course of action was to use a balloon, place it in the area of the plaque, expand it to push the plaque to the walls of the artery, and make more room for blood flow. If her arteries were significantly blocked, she could be referred to the surgeon for an open heart bypass. Helen's doctor chose to perform a balloon angioplasty – blow up the balloon in the area of her plaque, so an increased amount of blood could pass.

She returned to the floor with stable vitals. Within hours of the procedure, Helen began to complain of altered vision in her left eye and that her fingers and toes began to hurt. Her physical exam appeared normal. The doctor on for the evening shift sent her for a head CT scan. Labs were drawn. The doctor ran fluids, as her kidney function was a bit worse, which can be a side effect of the dye used for the procedure.

Helen's pain became worse. She also started developing a strange rash on her abdomen and legs. Her kidney function worsened in spite of fluids. Helen had experienced a cholesterol shower. This occurs when the plaque in her coronary artery came loose, and broke into microscopic pieces. These pieces lodged in the small capillaries in her fingers, toes, eyes, brain, and kidneys.

We gave Helen morphine to help ease her pain. This was way back before we had PCA pumps, or continuous morphine drips. I was in her room every hour, trying to keep this sweet woman comfortable, as she died. There was no treatment we had to cure this. As her capillaries became occluded with these plaques, and blood flow was cut off to the tissue, small wounds erupted on her skin. These wounds first appeared as dark, dry spots. Then they turned into wet, oozing areas – tens, if not one hundred of them – on her tiny body. The wounds became infected and had a unique odor. I later learned this was pseudomonas. In over thirty years, I've never forgotten that smell.

Helen died a peaceful death. She required increasing amounts of morphine to control her pain. She eventually was placed on a morphine drip. The infection got into her bloodstream and her blood pressure dropped dangerously low. Deciding against sending her to the ICU to be placed on machines, family made her comfortable. While Helen didn't get back to her house, her garden, her lunch dates, she was able to take her last breath with her family by her side.

## $\mathcal{I}$ IS FOR IODINE. $\mathcal{I}$ IS FOR INGUINAL HERNIA, INTUSSUSCEPTION, ICHTHYOSIS, AND IDIOPATHIC.

## $\mathcal{I}$ IS ALSO FOR IAN.

Ian was a 20-year-old male paraplegic. He grew up in a fatherless household. His mother worked to support Ian and his two siblings. There were times when she worked extra hours,well into the evening. When this happened, she would have Ian stay home to watch his younger brothers. As a teenager, he got angry. Ian didn't want to babysit. He wanted to be out with his friends. What teenager wants to be responsible for a 10 and 6-year-old? When his mother was home, he spent his evenings – sometimes until early in the morning – out with his buddies. They smoked, walked the streets, got high, stole. They certainly weren't up at all hours reading the Bible!

Eventually, his nighttime antics brought Ian to the police department. He wasn't put in jail, but now he was on their radar. Not only had he gotten the attention of the police, he had also been noticed by a local gang. Ian would make a nice addition to their posse. At first he resisted, but the more they encouraged him, taunted him, flaunted their guns, their money, their gang symbols, the more Ian became entranced. He snuck out of the house one midnight, and went to join the gang for his initiation.

This particular gang didn't beat him in. In order to prove his worth, Ian had to rob a convenience store, and shoot someone…not to kill, but to show he had the balls to pull a trigger. After scoping out a local 7-11, Ian put a plan together. He would enter the store about five minutes before it closed. With his mask to hide his face and his black clothes to help him disappear into the night, he would threaten the clerk with his pistol, and demand they give him all the money from the register. What Ian didn't figure into his plan was that there would be a friend of the clerk's in the store that night. When the clerk's friend heard the commotion, he pulled out his concealed gun and shot. The shot hit Ian, traveling through his left side, his spine, and resting just behind his right kidney. Ian hit the floor, paralyzed from the waist down.

I don't know the circumstances about his sentencing and jail time. What I do know is Ian's family did not want him to live his life in a nursing home, so they took him home. They promised they would take good care of him. Well….that didn't happen. He wasn't turned as he should have been, to relieve pressure on his body. His diet was junk (fast food,), so his body lacked the proper nutrients it needed to heal and rebuild.

By the time I met Ian, he had numerous deep ulcers on his buttocks, hips, even the insides and outside of his thighs and calves. This was the worst case of pressure wounds I had – and have – ever seen. The wounds were continuously getting infected, even causing sepsis. When this occurred, Ian was admitted to the ICU. I met him while working on our medical unit. At that time, Ian had been in the hospital for ten months. TEN MONTHS. His life had been a repeating cycle of ICU admit, transfer to the medical floor, get another infection, and back to the ICU. Through all of this, he somehow managed to escape being placed on a ventilator. The wound team had been consulted and gave orders on how to treat Ian's numerous wounds.

We were to clean the wounds with normal saline, place a damp dressing in some wounds, silvadene in others, cover with a dry dressing, and wrap the area in a gauze bandage. Some of the wounds, due to being in awkward locations, weren't wrapped in gauze, but covered in a type of dressing that looked like fishnet stockings. This dressing came in a stretchy, circular design. For the wounds on his hips, we would cut a large length of this tubular dressing, slide it up over both his legs, and it would end up going around both his hips. In order to change all of Ian's dressings, it would take between an hour and a half to two hours.. Also, our orders were to change the dressings twice a day. TWICE. When Ian was part of your patient assignment for the shift, you prayed your other patients would be pretty independent and not need much…of anything.

I have never been a psych nurse, but Ian's mental development, the way he interacted with staff, seemed to have been stunted. He spoke like a little child. I don't know if his dependence on his family, and eventually the medical staff, caused him to regress. I remember one shift, I was following a nurse named Mary. I had refused Ian something – I don't even remember what – to which he replied, "Well, Mawee let me do it." Not "Mary"… "Mawee."

The doctors had spoken to Ian about performing a pelvectomy. They would amputate at the level of his pelvis, which would involve removal of both hip joints. Ian would have a chest and abdomen – but nothing below. This would have required formation of a colostomy, and an ileal conduit, for his stool and urine to exit his abdomen. He was adamantly set against this. Even though his life was spent in bed, requiring assistance from others to turn, to sit up, to move, Ian would not let the doctors perform the surgery. He was born with two legs, and he was going to die with two legs.

And that's what Ian did. He became septic again. The doctors tried all they knew to do to save his life, but Ian had used up his ninth life. He died, with both his legs. All of this occurred because at sixteen, he was trying to prove how tough he was.

# *J* IS FOR JUGULAR. *J* IS FOR JOINT, JEJEUNUM, JUXTAPOSITION, AND JCAHO.

# *J* IS ALSO FOR JULIE.

Julie was a slender 56-year-old woman. She was married, had two grown children, and exercised five days a week. In fact, Julie had lost seventy-five pounds, and kept it off for two years. She promised herself that if she was able to keep the weight off for over just one year, she would have a breast lift.

During her first pregnancy, her weight gain was around fifty pounds. Julie's first child, a boy, was born in early September. Throughout that summer, her feet had become more swollen. She wore slippers in the house, and sandals outside. The swelling in her feet got so bad you could see the strap lines in her skin, hours after she took her sandals off. Not only did her feet get bigger, but so did her belly, and her breasts. By the end of her pregnancy, she was wearing bras two cup sizes bigger.

After the delivery, she returned to her pre-pregnancy weight. Her belly got smaller, and so did her breasts. Unfortunately, her breast tissue had been stretched so much, when she lost the weight, her breasts became a little saggy. Then came a second pregnancy – weight gain and breasts inflating and deflating like water balloons.

Julie bought all sorts of pretty, lacy bras to help hold her "girls" up. Until this time, I had never heard the term "girls". I'd heard "boobs", "bazingas", "tits", and all sorts of other terms, but not "girls". I remember having a conversation with Julie, and she was telling me about her "girls". "Oh. You have children," I asked. "No," Julie said. "My twins." "Oh" I replied. "You have twin girls?" Julie must have thought I was from outer space. " NO. MY BOOBS," she said emphatically. In my head I thought, *OH. Your BREASTS. Got it.*

The time came for Julie to ditch the pretty bras, and have her breast lift. She consulted a plastic surgeon, and the procedure was scheduled. The plan was to have her stay one night in the hospital. I cared for Julie in the late afternoon, following her surgery.

When I entered the room, her husband and mother were present. Julie was a bit sore, but the morphine was helping. Noted during my assessment were two drains, one exiting each upper breast. The tubing was approximately twelve inches long, attached to a small plastic drain shaped like a football. These drains were pinned to her hospital gown, to prevent them from falling out. We were to teach Julie how to empty these drains and record the amount coming from each. Her doctor would use this information at the post surgery visit, to determine when it was safe to pull the drains.

I was talking Julie through the process of emptying the first drain. I gently squeezed the drain as the drainage collected into a urine cup. These were used frequently due to their compact size, and measurement markings on the side of the container. I was looking for somewhere to place the urine cup, which was now filled with the warm, amber, blood-tinged drainage being produced by Julie's body. Her bedside table was full of items – her water pitcher and cup, glasses, and magazines. Thinking it would not be good technique to place this bodily fluid on the same table as her water, I set the cup on top of the vitals machine, next to her bed. As I was closing the clamp on her drain and pinning it back to her gown, I heard this whoosh.....................splat.

The next thing I knew, I was feeling this weird, warm sensation on my left leg and my lower abdomen. The top of the vitals machine wasn't perfectly flat. There was a bit of an angle. Who knew? My white scrub pants were now splattered with……. Julie. The drainage had splashed all over me … .and the floor, the wall, and the cupboards. I gasped, but managed to keep my cool. I wanted to start cleaning up this spill before I or anyone else slipped/ landed in the puddle of Julie. The first thing I found was a bath blanket. I threw it on the floor, and as I cleaned up the HAZMAT spill, I could feel Julie slowly running down my leg and into my sock and shoe. I had everything contained to the point I could now leave to call housekeeping, when Julie's mother got up out of her chair, walked over to where I was, pointed to the floor and said, "You missed a spot."

All I could think was, *Lady – I have your daughter dripping down my leg, and you dare tell me I missed a spot!!??* I just looked at her and said, "Yes. I know".

I left the room, and was able to get housekeeping to clean Julie's room. I was also able to get a change of clothes from surgery. Surgical scrubs always work in a pinch. I couldn't wait to get home and wash the Julie off my legs and out of my clothes.

# $\mathscr{K}$ IS FOR KILOGRAM. $\mathscr{K}$ IS FOR KIDNEY, KAWASAKI'S DISEASE, KERATECTOMY, AND KETONES.

# $\mathscr{K}$ IS ALSO FOR KEESHA.

Keesha was a 48-year-old black female I met while working in the ICU of a trauma center. She had a boyfriend named Bruce. Bruce and Keesha had been in a relationship for almost twenty years.

They both worked in the beginning. Whether out of excitement, curiosity, or boredom, they turned to drugs five years before I met them. At first, it was only on the weekends, a party here, a party there. When they became addicted, life got a lot harder. Keesha lost her job. Bruce managed to keep it together enough to do a half-assed job at the home improvement store where he worked in the lumber department. As more and more paychecks were spent on drugs, things like rent and food took a back seat. They would wait until dark, and go dumpster diving. One of the best places, Bruce told me, was behind a specialty grocery store. Once a week, Bruce and Keesha could find themselves feasting on unique items such as outdated gruyere cheese, imported Italian crackers, Greek olives, and maybe some prosciutto.

One night, while diving, Bruce came face-to-face with someone who wanted the food as badly as he and Keesha did – a big, fat raccoon. Before he could leap out of the dumpster, the varmint hissed, then lunged at him, biting him on his left calf. A phone call to a friend and he was in the ER within fifteen minutes. It was after

"

he completed the series of painful rabies shots that Bruce realized he had to make some changes. He quit the drugs cold turkey. He stayed home as Keesha took care of him, cleaning up his vomit if he missed the toilet. After five painful days, Bruce was through his withdrawal.

Keesha, however, was not. Though she was caring for Bruce, spooning chicken soup into his mouth, she was snorting coke up her nose. As Bruce's life was taking an upturn, Keesha's was spiraling downward. She became emotionally labile. When Bruce went to work, Keesha would stay home. She would do some coke, watch game shows, and pass out. She repeated this cycle in the afternoon, changing out heroin for the coke, and soap operas for game shows. If he was even just a few minutes late, Bruce knew there would be an argument. He may have just chatted with some coworkers after work, but in Keesha's mind, he was having an affair. In Keesha's mind, he was with someone prettier, thinner – someone clean.

One night Bruce had come home from work, and Keesha was not home. He enjoyed the quiet, no arguments, no accusations. When he woke up, he realized it was the next morning, and he was still alone in the house. Bruce began to panic as he called around to Keesha's friends, and no one knew where she was.

I knew where she was. I mean, eventually I knew. Overnight, we had a Jane Doe admitted to our ICU. We had a thin, young black woman who came in as a level 1 trauma, after she had been hit by a train. Witnesses told the police they saw a woman walk onto the tracks in the path of an oncoming train. At the last minute, they saw her head raise up.

Perhaps she was looking at the train? Maybe she changed her mind and was going to get up off the tracks. Either way, it was too late, and she was hit by the train. She was brought into the ER, an emergent orthopedic evaluation was requested, and she was taken to surgery. She had external fixators placed. An external fixator is a device which has screws placed into the bone, and a metal device is attached to the screws on the outside of the skin to help stabilize the broken bones. Jane Doe had an external fixator on each upper arm, thigh, and calf. Caring for these devices was tedious. There could be ten screws (pins) or more on each fixator. During every shift, we were to take Qtips and clean each pin with saline. Then we applied Bacitracin ointment. At times, it took one nurse to hold up a limb, and another to do the pin care.

I was finishing the pin care for my shift, when the nursing supervisor came into the room. She had a gentleman with her, whose wife was missing. He had heard about the train accident, and was wondering if Jane could actually be Keesha. We cleaned her up – she had been unresponsive for us since coming to the unit – and placed clean sheets on top of her, to make her look as presentable as we could make a woman with pounds of external hardware coming from each extremity. As we turned her to clean her, you could hear the clinkclinkclink of the fixators bumping against each other. We turned her to the other side – clinkclinkclink – and pulled the dirty sheets out from under her, and smoothed the clean ones. Coming into the room with the supervisor was a handsome gentleman, six feet tall, eyes red from crying. He took one look at Jane, and said, "Oh, my God. That's her." I had just met Bruce and Keesha.

We had Keesha in the unit for another forty-one days. She developed a GI bleed, and had to be scoped by GI. She also developed pneumonia and an ileus ( a portion of the small intestine that quits working), and had to have an NG tube placed through her nose into her stomach, hooked to suction so she wouldn't accumulate stomach contents and vomit. Over the weeks, Bruce came to see her less and less. He had contact information for her family, and while her mother was made her POA (power of attorney), she never came to visit. Eventually infection took over her body. Keesha's blood pressure began to drop. Her mother was called, and she stated she wanted us to make Keesha comfortable and let her go. Keesha's mother told us she had always been telling Keesha to stay away from drugs, or they would kill her.

Well, Keesha's mother was right. The drugs did lead to Keesha's death. Clinkclinkclink and all.

# $\mathscr{L}$ IS FOR LIP. $\mathscr{L}$ IS FOR LABIA, LUNG, LESION, AND LIPOMA.

# $\mathscr{L}$ IS ALSO FOR LINDA.

Linda was a 45-year-old-female who fit the three F's: fat, forty, and female. Those are some of the factors that predispose someone to gallstones.

Linda went to her doctor after she had been having nausea, vomiting, and right upper abdominal pain every time she ate for almost a month. She was happy she had been losing weight, but this is not how she wanted to do it. Scans showed Linda had a gallstone about the size of a marble, partially lodged in her common bile duct.

She was initially sent to a GI physician, for a procedure called an ERCP... Endoscopic retrograde cholangiopancreatography (mm-hmm...say that five times fast). An ERCP is a procedure in which the physician puts a scope through the patient's mouth, through the stomach, and into the first part of the small intestine. There, the physician then accesses the common bile duct, the pancreatic duct, and the gallbladder. Dye injected into these areas makes any stones (or other abnormalities) easier to visualize. In some cases, the physician is able to thread a small basket through the scope, grab the stone, and pull it out. This did not work in Linda's case. The stone was too large, and the physician was not comfortable attempting to pull this stone out, as it could cause considerable damage. Next step – surgery referral.

As luck would have it, Dr. Abe D. Omen was the surgeon on call that day. His caseload was light, so he agreed to take Linda to surgery. Three hours later, she arrived at my ambulatory surgery recovery unit. Her vitals were stable. She was sleepy from the anesthetic and the pain meds she was given in recovery (PACU), so I let her rest. There were three things we looked for in our patients to determine if they were ready to go home. Patients needed to walk without passing out, eat and drink (crackers and fizzy pop or water) without vomiting, and they needed to pee. Linda was able to eat her crackers, which she said tasted like heaven. The next step was to walk her to the bathroom, and see if she could urinate.

Now, let me go back to the beginning for a minute. Remember the fat, forty, and female? Again, Linda was all three. Also, she came up to my nose when another nurse and I were finally able to help her stand. When she was lying in the bed, I could barely fit two fingers between each of her hips and the side rails. I don't know how wide the beds are – but Linda was just as wide. There was no way I was going to walk her by myself. If she got weak or dizzy and started going down, all I would be able to do is watch.

We were able to get Linda into the restroom. It was the size of a half bath. When you opened the door, the toilet was on your right. Beyond the toilet was a very small shower. To your left was the sink. Once you stood up from the toilet, you could easily reach out and touch the sink. Linda was settled, so I closed the door almost all the way, and I stood outside the door. I never left my patients on the toilet unattended. One fall and splitting a scalp is one fall too many in my eyes. I would periodically give the "Linda, how ya' doing?" to which she would say, "I'm fine." The third time I asked, I heard, "Ok. I'm ready." I opened the door, and to my surprise, I saw Linda,

up off the toilet, leaning with her upper body over the sink. What???
I looked at her and said, "Linda? What are you doing?" Her reply? "I
need you to wipe me"........"You want me to …what?"

"Well, I cant reach. I can't do it myself. I need you to wipe me."
Now…all sorts of questions came flooding into my brain, including
the question of… *How does she do this at home if she can't reach?*
Maybe she knows Agatha!

I put the call light on as I grabbed the wipes. Yes. I wiped
Linda. When the other nurse arrived, we walked Linda back to bed.
It's never easy to get someone in the perfect position when they get
back in bed. They end up at the bottom of the bed, with the draw
sheet halfway up their back. Or, they end up on their backs, right up
against a side rail (or any other several crooked ways). There was no
way two of us were going to be able to straighten her up, even with
the draw sheet. With assistance from our nursing assistant, the three
of us were able to pull Linda up in bed.

Linda made a successful recovery. We were able to take out her
IV, help her get dressed, and turn her over to the care of her husband
to drive her home. We put her discharge instructions, her plastic
water glass, her bra (I don't blame her) in her patient belongings bag
to take home with her. Oh…and the wipes. Definitely the wipes.

## *M* IS FOR MUSCLE. *M* IS FOR MYOPATHY, METHEMOGLOBIN, MYASTHENIA GRAVIS, AND MAGGOTS.

## *M* IS ALSO FOR MELODY.

Melody (Mel, to her family) was a 24-year-old female I met in a respiratory care unit. She had been transferred to us from another hospital so we could manage her trach, a hole cut in the front of her neck, with a plastic tube inserted into her trachea (windpipe) to allow her to breathe. Mel also had a tube in her abdomen that connected with her stomach. This allowed us to feed her, because she was not able to swallow on her own. She would be receiving intense physical and occupational therapy over the next few weeks. Mel would be learning how to walk, how to dress and feed herself, and how to use a toilet normally. Why, you ask, does a 24-year-old need all these things? Well…

Mel had begun running a fever and not feeling well, while she was away at college. She didn't think it was serious, so she fought on. She went to class for a few hours one morning, where she developed abdominal pain and vomiting. Mel called her mother while a friend drove her to the ER. Labs and a CT scan of her abdomen revealed she had appendicitis. Although she was old enough to sign her own consents, Mel did not want to do anything until her mother could get to the hospital. The drive from home to the hospital would take almost an hour. The ER physician called in a surgery consult. The surgeon wanted to take Mel to the operating room right away, but she wouldn't budge until mom arrived.

Mom made it to the hospital. Mel's pain was increasing, and the surgeon was becoming more insistent they get to OR, even telling Mel she could die if her appendix were to burst. Paperwork was done, mom got a quick kiss on the cheek, and Mel was off to surgery. The surgeon made his entry into the abdomen, and as he touched the appendix and prepared to remove it, it burst like a squeezed pimple. Infection spread into her abdomen, and Mel's "routine" surgery suddenly became not so routine. Now her abdomen had to be irrigated to remove as much of the infection as possible. To make matters worse, while cleaning out her abdomen – the surgeon nicked an artery. The bleeding was difficult to control. What seemed like eternity took minutes to get stopped.

It wasn't until she was not waking up as expected in the recovery room that something was noticeably wrong. Blood gases were checked, labs drawn, and a head CT was done. Instead of waking up and going home, Mel was transferred to the ICU. Neurology was consulted. It was determined Mel suffered an anoxic (loss of oxygen) brain injury in surgery. She had bled so much her brain suffered lack of blood flow, which also meant lack of oxygen supply. Mel had to be on the ventilator (breathing machine) for a prolonged period of time. In fact, she needed to be on the ventilator so long, instead of being connected to a tube that was inserted through her mouth and into her lungs, she had the tracheostomy surgically placed. The tube through the mouth was removed, and she was attached to the ventilator via this tube in her neck. Mel was eventually able to breathe on her own, but because she was so weak, the trach was left in place to protect her airway.

Mel's light red wavy hair and her freckles reminded me of my own child. She had a slim build. Her mom and sister took turns painting her finger and toenails. Her mom brought in her favorite pillow and blanket from home. On either side of her, she liked to have her stuffed animals placed under her arms, so she could feel them when she woke up. Her favorites were two brightly colored butterflies. Mel's mother explained to us Mel was very close to her grandmother – her father's mother. Nana, as Mel called her, baked cookies, taught Mel how to sew, and how to care for flowers in her garden. Occasionally they would be visited by butterflies. According to Nana, this was a sign that no matter how things were in the world, no matter how bad everything seemed, it would all turn out alright.

We had Mel on our unit for almost four weeks. With therapy, she got stronger. She had speech therapy work with her to learn how to swallow again. It was just a couple of days before she left us that she began taking sips of water and eating a soft diet. The plan was to make sure Mel was able to eat solid food, get enough calories each day, and the feeding tube in her abdomen would be removed. We were slowly replacing the breathing tube in her neck with smaller sizes. She would see a doctor after she was discharged who would remove the tube permanently, and observe her as the hole in her neck healed shut.

Six months later, I was working a Saturday on the unit. A pretty redhead walked up to our nurses' desk carrying three boxes, each containing a dozen cupcakes. She looked familiar, but I couldn't place how I knew her. She set the boxes down. "May I help you?" I asked. A big grin came across her face, as she reached up and pulled the upper part of her shirt to the left, revealing a beautiful tattoo of a butterfly, resting just over her heart. Under the tattoo, in elegant script, was tattooed the word – Nana.

# *N* IS FOR NOSE. *N* IS FOR NARCAN, NARCISSIST, NARCOLEPSY, AND NECROTIZING FASCIITIS.

# *N* IS ALSO FOR NATHAN.

Nathan, or Nate, as he was called by his parents, was a 46-year-old biomedical technician. His job was to maintain and repair the vital equipment used in the hospital – everything from IV pumps, blood pressure machines, and monitors in the ICU. His parents told us he was a loving son. He would check on them every day, and even stop by on his days off. He was funny, intelligent, and loved dogs. He was also morbidly obese. Nate weighed over five hundred pounds.

Nate had no shortage of friends, male and female. What he didn't have was a successful love life. His mother stated Nate had been interested in a few women throughout his life. Due to his weight, she believed, a serious relationship never developed. He never had problems finding a dinner date, a movie date, someone to have coffee with. When he got up the nerve to express his deep feelings for a woman, somehow they would manage to disappear. Nate's mother told us one way he dealt with his feelings was to eat. He preferred sweets, and he knew the best bakeries in town. Greek baklava, Boston cream pie from Indulge, and chocolate cream pie from Betty's were some of his favorites.

Three weeks before I met Nate and his parents, another woman in Nate's life gave him the "just friends" speech. Nate's mother told us he had developed strong feelings for a woman he met at the local dog park. Nate would take Bitsy, his eight pound mutt he rescued from a shelter. Many nights he would see Marcia there, with her fifty pound pitbull mix, Tuffy. While Bitsy and Tuffy would play, Marcia and Nate would slowly walk the perimeter of the dog park, chatting about their work, their day, their lives. Nate got up the nerve one evening to tell Marcia he was falling in love with her. Nate's mother stated after that, he never saw Marcia again at the dog park.

Nate's parents became worried when they had not heard from him in two days. It was not like him to go so long without reaching out to them. Nate's father tried to call, and when he didn't get an answer on the other end of the phone, he drove to Nate's house. There, he saw something he will never forget. He found Nate lying in his bathtub, a scimitar ( a sword with a curved blade) sticking out of his abdomen. Nate had brought this sword home with him after a trip to Japan two years ago. Now it was off his wall, the instrument he used to try to kill himself.

I was walking back to the ICU after my lunch break. The exterior of the hospital was composed of a multitude of windows. It was enjoyable returning to my unit this way, as this was the only way some days I knew if it was sunny, if it had snowed, if it was day or night. This path would take me by the helipad, where the trauma patients were rushed off the helicopters and into the ER. This particular day I stopped in my tracks, unsure what I was seeing. The medic crew was pushing a gurney. On the gurney was a figure covered with blankets – blankets that seemed to be piled 3 feet high. Later, I learned this was Nate. The medics brought him in, sword in place. They knew not to pull it out, as Nate could bleed internally, and possibly die before he made it to the hospital.

Nate had an extremely rough hospital course. He was taken to surgery that day. It was a long surgery, as the damage internally was extensive. Most swords are straight, causing a linear path of damage. A scimitar, however, is curved. As Nate plunged the sword into his abdomen, it had caused an arc of destruction. After surgery, he came to the ICU. The surgeon told us he left Nate's abdomen open. He would plan on taking Nate back to surgery, two more times, in order to allow adequate healing. The fact there was a foley catheter to drain his bladder, a colostomy to drain stool externally as his colon was damaged, a central line – a large IV line in a vein in his neck – was no surprise to us.

Nate was kept sedated, and on a ventilator. The plan was to allow him to wake up after his third surgery, as long as things were going as planned. Unfortunately, Nate developed pneumonia. Then he developed a high fever, and the infectious disease doctor determined Nate had developed an abscess ( a pocket of infection) in his abdomen. Due to the complications, he needed to be on the ventilator for a prolonged period of time. While patients are on the ventilator, a tube is inserted through the mouth into the lungs. The tube can cause irritation over time. For patients who need continued ventilator support, the tube is removed, and a tracheostomy is placed in the front of the neck. This is a shorter tube that enters the airway, and the ventilator is then attached to this tube.

At this time, I was working weekends in the unit. I returned one Saturday, and Nate was not in the unit. Of course, I inquired as to where he was. The nurses told me Nate had his third surgery, and he also had the tracheostomy placed. During a weaning trial, where the sedation is decreased to allow a patient to start waking up, Nate had become restless. He would keep violently shaking his head side to side. The nurses upped his sedation again to help calm him down. His ventilator kept alarming. Connections and settings were checked. After some time had passed, it was discovered Nate had dislodged the trach from his airway. It was no longer in the airway, but sitting under the skin of his neck. Nate was so obese and his neck so large, it was difficult to see this. By the time it was discovered, Nate had been without a source of oxygen for approximately twenty minutes. He suffered an anoxic brain injury (brain damage from lack of oxygen). His parents had made the decision to remove him from life support the day before I returned to work.

As a way of thanking the team for caring for Nate, his parents sent us food – Greek baklava, Boston cream pie, and chocolate cream pie.

# *O* IS FOR OBTUNDED. *O* IS FOR OXYGEN, OBTURATOR, ORTHOPEDICS, AND OBSTIPATION.

# *O* IS ALSO FOR OSCAR.

Oscar was a very sweet 27-year-old male from Ecuador. His parents, two sisters and one brother, all immigrated to the U.S. when Oscar was twelve. Oscar spoke English well, albeit with an accent.

During our conversations, he would talk about his childhood – how he would give his food to his siblings so they would not go hungry, while he went to bed many nights, stomach growling. Oscar would walk with his younger sister to and from school in order to make sure she was not kidnapped, sold for drugs, or sex trafficked. Three years older than him, Oscar's brother was beginning to run with a bad crowd. They would steal whatever they could, and sell the items on the street for money. Unfortunately, the money did not go to the family. His brother would spend the money on clothes, on "bling", as Oscar called it. Fearing he would end up dead or in jail, his parents moved the family to the United States.

Also during our conversations, a sitter was present in Oscar's room. You see, Oscar was suffering from mental illness. Mental illness can begin to show itself in the teen years. Oscar's mother told us Oscar used to mumble under his breath, as if he was talking to himself. He would stare off in space, nodding his head, as if he was communicating with someone only he could see. Angry outbursts were nearly a daily occurrence. His doctor started him on medication, but it was difficult to get Oscar to take it every day. Then Oscar began swallowing things.

The endoscopy team at the hospital was familiar with him. When Oscar began to complain of his stomach hurting, his mother knew she had to get him to the hospital. He was known to have marbles, screws, even ketchup packets and a small crucifix in his stomach – all retrieved during an endoscopic procedure. This involved sedating him, the physician inserting a scope through his throat into his stomach. The physician then ran a pair of forceps down the scope, grabbing onto the object in Oscar's stomach, and slowly pulling back the scope until it was all the way out of the mouth. Then the physician would release whatever object they retrieved, insert the scope again, and this would continue until Oscar's stomach was empty of foreign objects.

To prevent this from happening in the hospital, Oscar was under constant surveillance. It was the sitter's job to make sure, even when he slept, his hands were visible at all times. Oscar could move quickly, and if you were distracted, suddenly his hands were up by his mouth. I had even heard from a nurse who cared for him at a previous admission. She had lost a pen. It was eventually found, just a small portion protruding from the tip of Oscar's penis (and no, I have no idea how it was found – or how it got there!).

I enjoyed caring for Oscar. He was a sweet, funny, cute, smart, mentally ill young man. Or I should say, a sweet, funny, cute, smart young man who just happened to have a mental illness. He would always give the "Yes, ma'am" or "No, ma'am." His teeth were straight and white, giving him a beautiful smile.

About a year after I last saw him, I learned Oscar had died. His mother had been urged by staff many, many times to place Oscar in a mental health facility. She refused. Her thought, as I've seen on multiple occasions with multiple patients, was that her job was to care for Oscar at home, and when he ran into trouble, it was our job to fix him. He was in the hospital again, being taken to radiology by two staff members, when he managed to undo a screw from the cart, and swallow it. Unfortunately, it lodged in his esophagus, causing a tear. This was not discovered right away. Oscar eventually needed surgery to repair the tear, but he developed several complications, and died.

Mental illness is a bitch. It can take some sweet, wonderful people and turn them into sweet, wonderful, time consuming, energy consuming, exhausting people.

Bitch.

$\mathscr{P}$ **IS FOR PERFORATE.** $\mathscr{P}$ **IS ALSO FOR PODIATRIST, PALPABLE, PANCREAS, AND PANDEMIC.**

$\mathscr{P}$ **IS ALSO FOR PIERRE.**

Pierre was a plump, African male whom I encountered on many occasions. He accompanied several of the clinic's African patients on their office visits. The African community in the area was very close knit; they looked out for one another. They knew Pierre by name, and he often drove them to the provider appointments.

When I had to perform a prostate exam on a male, Pierre gave a thorough explanation, in their native language (at least, I assumed he was explaining things to them!). On one occasion, I had the dreaded task of telling a family their loved one was going to die. He cried with us.

I remember a patient who only came to see me twice in three years. She was a 48 – year-old female with uncontrolled hypertension. More than once she came in, and we rechecked her blood pressure three times because we could not believe she was actually 247/130. She would deny any chest pain, headaches, shortness of breath. My challenge with this particular patient was she also had severe mental illness. She was a paranoid schizophrenic. I tried everything to explain to her why she needed to take her medications, but all she would say to me in English was " I'm fine." I could not get her to let us draw her labs. I was extremely worried about the condition of her heart and kidneys. Pierre tried to help me explain these things to her.

As we talked, the patient would say "Yah, yah." I thought that meant she understood. I learned that it actually means "No." I was telling the patient why she needed blood pressure medicine, and she was saying "Yah, yah." I thought, *Great, she understands,* " when in fact she was telling me "No, no."

I asked Pierre one day if he knew anything about the patient's background, if she suffered from mental illness her entire life. Here is what he told me: Maria – I'll call her Maria – was born and grew up in Africa. She was married, and had four children, and became pregnant with her fifth. When the government began killing its own citizens, Maria and her family fled to a refugee camp. Unfortunately, the government soldiers made their way to the camps. Maria saw her own children get tortured. She witnessed the soldiers cutting off her children's hands, killing them. She herself was raped, and stabbed, causing her to lose the baby. Maria had not been the same since.

As he was telling me this, I kept opening my eyes wider, trying to keep tears from running down my cheeks. *I'm the practitioner,* I thought. *I have to be the strong one.* Finally, I couldn't control it any longer, and I gave in to my tears. I reached for the nearest paper towel – I was out of Kleenex – and wiped the tears and snot from my face. I could not believe what I was hearing.

I hate getting stuck in traffic behind someone actually driving the speed limit. I get frustrated when the local donut shop is out of my cream filled long johns. I hate having to dodge someone else's dog crap when I walk my dog.

First world problems, for sure. For sure.

# $\mathcal{Q}$ IS FOR QUADRANTS. $\mathcal{Q}$ IS FOR QUADRICEPS, QUININE, QUADRIPLEGIA, AND QRS COMPLEX.

# $\mathcal{Q}$ IS ALSO FOR QUEEN.

Seriously. She told us all to call her "Queen".

Queen was a morbidly obese 50-something black woman. She used phrases like "You know it, girl" and "My momma would whoop my ass if I did/said something like that. Mm-hmm". Her nails were brightly colored, looking like daggers coming off the tip of her fingers. Before it was trendy, she had those fake, Bambi eyelashes. Queen loved her children. I would hear her call them in the evening as her husband, at home, was getting them ready for bed. "Momma loves you. I'll be home soon".

We admitted Queen as a patient after she had gone to see her doctor for what she thought was severe allergies. She told us her skin was so dry, no lotion helped. She would scratch and scratch until she bled. No over the counter medications helped and she was hoping her doctor would prescribe her something.

Even though Queen had diabetes and high blood pressure, she didn't always take her medications like she should. "Why should I put all that in my body when I feel fine?" she would ask. How many times have we heard that? Queen would take her blood pressure medicine for a while. Magically, at her office visits, her blood pressure would be controlled – so she would stop the medications again. "See – my blood pressure is fine now."

This time, things were not fine. Queen's doctor sent her to the ER for a blood pressure of 240/120. How she did not have a raging headache is beyond me. She also had labs done. Her diabetic marker – her A1c – was over 11. It should be less than 7. Her kidney markers showed her kidneys were in failure. Stage 4, to be exact (in kidney stages, 1 is great; 5 means you need dialysis…again, Queen was in stage 4). The kidney specialists (nephrology) had been consulted. They were managing her meds as best they could in the hopes of bringing her kidney function up. Stage 3 was the goal. Insulin was ordered by endocrinology (the diabetes gurus) to get her blood sugars under tight control. Queen didn't like all the pokes, but when you started discussing toe amputations, eyesight loss, and dialysis – she didn't mind the pokes so much.

I worked the 11pm to 7am shift. Queen was so excited. She told me her kidney function was getting better, and she had been scared enough "this time" that she was more motivated to take care of herself when she got home. She was going to have labs drawn in the following morning. If her kidney function had improved enough, the nephrologists might let her go home.

I gave Queen's report to the oncoming day shift nurse, and sat down to finish my charting.

The phlebotomist – the person who draws blood, the "Vampire" as they get called – came to me and told me she couldn't wake up the patient in room three. Holy shit! Queen's room.

I ran into her room and found Queen lying on her back, snoring. Had I ever noticed that she snores? I tried as hard as I could, but she would not wake up. A code blue was called. After what seemed an eternity – actually just under fifteen minutes – the physician running the code called an end to it. Queen was in PEA – pulseless electrical activity. The electricity was running though her heart, but the pump of the heart was not responding. She was dead.

A few weeks later, I heard that her autopsy revealed that an aneurysm in the large artery in her abdomen had ruptured. She bled to death, internally.

I miss our nighttime chats, her laugh. I miss hearing her say, "Momma loves you. I'll be home soon".

Long live the Queen.

# *R* IS FOR RABIES. *R* IS FOR RADIATION, RNA, REFLUX, AND REFLEX.

# *R* IS ALSO FOR RAKISHA.

Rakisha was in my unit because she had a wound that needed to be managed, and she could not manage it herself at home.

Let me 'splain, Lucy.

Snorting heroin was her vice. Rakisha didn't drink, she didn't shop, and she wasn't a clothes fiend. She was a woman in her fifties who didn't work. She was on disability due to back pain she suffered after a fall from a forklift at work, five years previously. At first, physical therapy and some hydrocodone helped her pain. It also gave her the "whoo-hoo"s. Rakisha started liking the "hydrobuzz" as she called it. She would think of different reasons to see her doctor – all of them pain related – so she could get more hydrocodone. Eventually, her doctor told her he was no longer going to order any narcotics for her.

This led to a series of ER visits, all related to pain complaints. Rashika got flagged as a drug seeker. She was burning up all her bridges.

Unable to obtain any more hydrocodone, she would ask her friends, even people she didn't know – if they could supply her with something to replace her hydrobuzz. This is when she started taking anything she could get her hands on – cocaine, methadone, and heroin. Heroin became her favorite. She called it her "love". It never let her down.

Rashika's favorite way to indulge was to smoke it. She told me she enjoyed not only the buzz, but the process… the preparation of the foil, the heating up of the heroin. To her it was like Christmas Eve – she knew something enjoyable was just around the corner.

When she wasn't doing her heroin, Rashika enjoyed being a grandma. Her son had a 5 year-old that she spoiled like crazy. She enjoyed spending time with him, hearing him call her "Nana". She enjoyed watching him spill Spaghettios in her kitchen. She loved his giggle while playing in the bathtub. Her daughter's pregnancy and upcoming due date had HER giggling. Rashika couldn't wait to be a grandma to a little girl.

Now…back to her wound.

For some reason she couldn't explain, Rashika decided one day she didn't want to smoke her heroin. She wanted to inject it. So she did. The buzz was like no other, she told me, like an orgasm for your brain. As high as it made her, soon after, she would begin to experience a terrible low. Rashika was a black woman. Dark skin. She knew something was wrong when she started to feel like she was getting the flu – and she noticed a dark line start to creep from the injection site up her arm. It became painful. When she started to throw up, her daughter brought her to the ER.

Rashika had developed an infection that was spreading into her bloodstream. She was given an IV, and started on antibiotics. She felt like crap for almost a week, and then her condition began improving. Her nausea went away; her fever came down. Rashika thought she was in the clear. Unfortunately, her arm started to swell… and swell. She had some residual infection in her arm the antibiotics hadn't cleared. The only way to save her arm was for a surgeon to make an incision in her forearm, almost down to the muscle, and leave that part of her arm open – not sutured shut. A wound vac was placed.

This was a cushioned pad placed right into the open area in Rashika's arm. A plastic dressing attached to a hose was placed on top. The other end of the hose was attached to a vacuum, kind of like a Foodsaver for your limb. This would provide constant suction to the wound, sucking out any drainage that could possibly lead to another infection. This whole dressing set up was changed about every three days.

One of my weekend shifts with Rashika was spent going into her room almost every hour. If the seal on the dressing was broken, the machine would stop, and beep at us to let us know it needed attention. I would try to patch her dressing as well as I could to maintain the suction, and an hour later I was back in her room. This particular time, it looked like a rat had been scratching at the dressing. It was itching, she told me, so she was scratching and picking at it.

I'm not usually a nurse who expresses my frustration at work, but something this day just tripped my trigger. I was very firm with her – I didn't yell – but I told her if she didn't quit picking, her arm was never going to heal. I told her she was at risk of another bad infection, and if we couldn't heal her arm, she could lose her arm. Then I said, "And how are you going to pick up your grandbabies with one arm?"

Something must have sunk in because her machine didn't beep again for the rest of my shift.

I was working weekends at that time and had been off for a week. When I returned to work, another nurse had Rashika as a patient. I didn't see her my whole 12-hour shift. Getting ready to leave at almost midnight, Rashika came up to me. My first thought was, "Uh-oh. What's up?" Rashika told me she wanted to thank me. "You're the only one who yelled at me," she said. Again, I promise, I had not yelled. "I didn't like it, but I needed to hear it." She explained that hearing me ask her how she could lift her grandkids with only one arm hit home for her. Those grandkids were her world. She realized if she didn't get her act together, she might not live to see them grow up. She quit picking at her dressing, and her arm healed well enough the wound vac could be removed. With continued dressing care, it healed completely. Rashika even gave me a hug that night.

She never returned to our unit, and as far as I know, she was not a patient in the hospital again. I had heard she was enjoying those grandkids – proudly tossing them up in the air – with two arms.

# $\mathscr{S}$ IS FOR SUTURE. $\mathscr{S}$ IS FOR SALMONELLA, SYNCOPE, SPLEEN, AND SCIATICA.

# $\mathscr{S}$ IS ALSO FOR SABRINA.

Sabrina was a 27-year-old patient I saw in the clinic. Only once. But she is forever ingrained in my memory, as is her baby girl.

As I was getting ready to enter the exam room, my medical assistant gave me a brief report on my patient: a 27-year-old female, eight months pregnant, did not speak English, and developed a right facial droop about a week ago. Sabrina had walked into our clinic a couple of days ago, but was told we had no openings, and she would have to come back. And here she was. In my exam room. Pregnant. Holy crap.

The translator and I met with Sabrina. I asked her all the questions I knew to ask. When did it start? Are there issues anywhere besides the face? How long does the droop last throughout the day?... all my OLDCARTS questions. While speaking with Sabrina, I asked my medical assistant to have our office physician come to the room. I was quietly trying not to freak out. We were blessed to have a very kind OBGYN also in our clinic, so I asked that he come in as well. And there we were – me, the two clinic MDs, the translator, and the patient all in a tiny exam room. Did I mention she was PREGNANT ?!

"Raise your eyebrows." She raised her eyebrows. "Smile." She smiled. "Close your eyes and don't let me pull them open." Every test we performed, Sabrina complied. Did she really raise both eyebrows the same? "Raise them again for me." Was her smile really symmetrical? "Smile again for me." It seemed there was a subtle weakness on the right side of her face. The OBGYN by now had left the room. "I don't know nothin' about strokes – I just birth babies." The other physician, who was not only a kind, gentle soul but also my collaborative physician, felt the patient was experiencing Bell's palsy. Bell's palsy is a condition that affects the nerve controlling one side of the face, causing muscle weakness. Typically, this was treated with antiviral medication and steroids. Through the translator, I explained my plan to Sabrina. Medications were sent to her pharmacy, and the medical assistant gave her a copy of her patient plan. This was right before lunch.

Prior to becoming a NP, I was an admission nurse in a local hospital. If you were going to be admitted, I was the gal who asked you a ton of questions you didn't feel well enough to answer at the time. Much of my time was spent in the ER as that was where the majority of our admitted patients came from. I tried to watch the ER providers as much as I could. What questions did they ask? What orders did they give? When a code stroke was called, as the paramedics were wheeling the patient through the ER doors, the provider would go right up to the gurney, perform an exam, and off the patient went to get a CT scan of the head. I watched as the provider had the patient smile, raise their eyebrows, frown, and close their eyes tightly. I remembered those times, and I couldn't stop thinking about Sabrina – and her baby. What if it wasn't Bell's palsy but something more serious? What if she indeed had a stroke? It wasn't just her that would be affected, but her unborn baby. Over lunch I scrolled through as many books as possible. I did searches on Bells palsy vs. stroke. My collaborative physician was my mentor, my guide, but at the end of the day, it was my name on Sabrina's chart.

I had the translator call Sabrina and have her go to the ER. I called the ER and gave her report to one of the physicians, asking him to get a CT scan of her head. If everything was normal, we would have wasted just a bit of her time.

As we were wrapping up our day in the office, I received a call from the ER. I thought the ER doc was just giving me a courtesy call to tell me Sabrina's head CT was negative. I must have looked shocked, as my collaborative physician asked me what was wrong. Sabrina's head CT showed she had a tumor that was pressing on her internal carotid artery. She was transferred directly from the ER to our university high risk OB center about ninety miles away. My higher power was definitely on my shoulder that day. So was Sabrina's!

Sabrina did not have surgery but she was watched very closely. She would alternate OB visits between the OB in our office, and the high risk center. I learned later that she had a normal delivery, and she and the baby were doing fine. The doctors felt that once she delivered the baby and lost some of her pregnancy fluid, the pressure would be lifted off the carotid artery.

One day soon after, I was standing at my usual spot in the office, just a few feet from the exam rooms, and a short hallway down from the OB's exam rooms. I saw a woman walk through, holding a tiny baby – and it was Sabrina, coming for her postpartum visit. Our eyes met and we smiled at each other. I don't know if she remembered me, but I sure knew who she was.

I am so grateful that I listened to my gut the day Sabrina appeared in my exam room. So f*#&ing grateful.

$\mathcal{T}$ **IS FOR TEST TUBE.** $\mathcal{T}$ **IS FOR TESTICLES, TARSALS, TETANUS, AND TELOMERE.**

$\mathcal{T}$ **IS ALSO FOR THERESA.**

Theresa had been married to Ralph for nearly seventy ears. He was definitely her soulmate. When Ralph developed a cough and started to feel run down, he – as most men – told her it would go away. Seeking medical treatment was not something he routinely did. The majority of time he went to see a provider was when he got tired of Theresa nagging him.

When he presented to our ER, it was because he got tired of hearing the "Ralph, you'd better go see the doctor" recording, over and over and……over. He figured he'd get some medicine, maybe an antibiotic, and he would be allowed to go home. What Ralph did not figure on was the ER nurses being more concerned about Theresa than they were him.

Theresa was pale, weak, and appeared to be having trouble breathing, as she was trying to tell the nurses about Ralph. One concerned nurse put a pulse ox probe on Theresa's frail finger. This was to read the oxygen level in her blood. The highest the probe can read is 100%. We like to see it read at least 90%. Theresa's level was 84%. This was an indication she was not getting enough oxygen in her blood, and therefore not enough oxygen to her major organs, including her heart, her kidneys, and her brain. When I was called to the ER to admit a patient, it wasn't Ralph I was admitting, but Theresa.

She was, as we found out, COVID positive. As I maneuvered through our hospital for over a year during the peak of COVID, we could never, with 100% certainty, predict how someone would progress through the disease. I saw 70-year-olds I thought would never come off a ventilator, sitting up on a cart and saying goodbye to us as the EMT crew took them to a skilled facility where they would get therapy to get stronger before they returned home. I saw 50-year – olds spend weeks on a ventilator as we saw their lungs get progressively worse on daily Xrays. We flipped them, back to stomach and back again, day after day. We inserted more tubes in them and called university hospitals to see if they had anything to offer the patient we were not. Those ICU physicians told us we were treating patients the same way they would – and, oh – one other thing. They were full and had no beds in their hospital for their own ER patients, let alone a transferred patient.

Theresa required increasing amounts of oxygen over the next several days. She still had an alert mind, and when we had some difficult discussions, she told me she did not want to go on a ventilator. If things got that bad, she just wanted us to keep her comfortable until she died. Through this, we were calling and updating her family. Even as Theresa was declining, her children would not come to the hospital to see her. They were all deathly afraid of catching COVID (although I suspect one of them may have been the reason she caught it in the first place). One child who was deathly afraid of catching COVID couldn't come to the hospital – because they were going on vacation to visit family and attend a school graduation. Umm…yeah. Don't get me started.

I was off on a weekend, and on Monday I went to check on Theresa. The floor nurse caught me and told me Theresa had a roommate now – Ralph. What??? Ralph had been sent home the day he was seen in ER.

Ralph had continued to get worse at home, however, getting more short of breath, weaker. He now needed oxygen himself, although not the high levels we were giving Theresa. The nurses had decided since they were a couple, and both COVID positive, they put Ralph in the same room as Theresa. Oh – did I forget to mention – surprise! Ralph was also COVID positive. He had tested positive in the ER, but because his oxygen level was normal, he had been allowed to go home.

Theresa continued to decline. At night, the nurses would push their beds together so they could hold hands. I was not due at work for a couple of hours when one of the floor nurses called me. Theresa had taken a turn for the worse. The nurses called the family, who still refused to come to the hospital. We had previously told them we would dress them up just as we did – gowns, gloves, masks, face shields – but they still refused. For the approximately fourteen days she was in the hospital, Theresa's children never came to see her. Not once. The nurse told me she was afraid Theresa would die alone. Yes, Ralph was there. He was ill himself, though, and there were times he didn't seem to understand how ill his wife was. I gathered my things and drove to the hospital.

When I arrived, I had to put my protective gear on, head to knees. It was not my preferred way to sit with a dying patient, but it's what had to be done at the time. I said hello to Ralph, and pulled a chair up to Theresa's bed. She was no longer responsive. As I sat with her, I held her hand. Her breathing became more irregular. Deep, then shallow..then none. There would be a deep inhalation, and the pattern would start all over. Through this, Ralph would ask me how she was doing. I would tell him she appeared comfortable. The nurses had already pushed the beds together so he could hold her hand.

I was with them for about twenty minutes, when Ralph got a call. It was one of his children. As he spoke to them, I noticed Theresa's breathing slowing. Twelve breaths a minute to six…then four….then….none. I heard Ralph tell his child he would call them back later and I jumped in – "Wait,wait,wait. Ralph. Don't hang up. She's gone." There may have been a more eloquent way to tell him this, but in that moment, that's what came out. "Oh," he said. To the person on the phone, "Well, I guess she is gone." Very matter-of – factly. I wondered if Ralph had been some type of engineer in his life – pencil pushing, pocket protector wearing, unemotional numbers guy. "Yes. I'm sorry," I said. "She has died."

Once the floor nurse was notified, they offered to move Ralph to a different room so he wouldn't have to be in there with all the post death activity. Ralph chose to stay with her until the time the funeral home came to pick her up. I had to move on to my other patients.

I later visited Ralph. He seemed to be in good spirits. He was dealing with his wife's death in his own way. One thing I still struggle with is realizing not everyone reacts the same. Some people wail and throw themselves on the floor when a loved one dies. Some people don't shed a tear. Ralph was not a tear shedder.

Four days later, Ralph was doing well enough that he was able to be discharged home. He would have visiting nurses to keep an eye on him for several weeks. I assume his family returned from vacation, but I never heard if they went to his home in the following weeks to check on him as well. The fact he was able to go home, at his age, after COVID, made him one of the lucky ones. The very lucky ones.

# $\mathcal{U}$ IS FOR ULTRASOUND. $\mathcal{U}$ IS FOR ULNA, UREA, URETER, AND UVEITIS.

# $\mathcal{U}$ IS ALSO FOR URSELA.

Ursela was a 56-year-old woman who loved farming and macaroni and cheese – homemade, of course. She loved her three children. She and her husband raised them to be honest, kind, and hardworking. Her two sons were planning on staying physically close when they graduated from high school so they could continue to help with the farm.

Her 8-year-old daughter wasn't sure if she wanted to be an astronaut, a veterinarian, or a chef. Patty Jo, or PJ as her family called her, enjoyed spending time with her mom. Ursela didn't do anything outer space related, but PJ still dreamed. PJ saved the money she was given for her birthday so she could buy food for the dogs and cats at the animal shelter. She loved helping out in the kitchen and dropping off food to the homeless.

It was PJ's dream that prompted Ursela and her husband to enroll PJ in Space Camp, in Huntsville, Alabama. Huntsville is a mere six hundred miles from their home. Because of his work schedule, Ursela and her husband decided Ursela would drive PJ to Alabama. PJ's dad would fly down a few days later, and they would drive back home together.

PJ helped her mom pack food for the road. She included some of her "gourmet" PB&J sandwiches – peanut butter, marshmallow cream, and Cheerios. Mmmm. I'll take two, please. Ursela packed the suitcases, threw them in the car, and off they went on a grand adventure.

It WAS grand, until….

As energetic and bubbly as she was, Ursela was NOT a very experienced highway driver. Growing up on farms, her driving consisted mostly of maneuvering the riding lawn mower and driving the pickup to get loads of hay. As she and PJ traversed some unfamiliar, winding two lane roads, Ursela approached a curve at a speed higher than the speed limit sign suggested. She rounded the curve and found herself in the lane of oncoming traffic. She swerved, the oncoming car swerved, yet they crashed into each other. Her driver's side front panel and door absorbed the impact – as did Ursela's body – and her head.

I don't know the specifics, but somehow Ursela's husband was able to get her transferred to our ICU. She was on a ventilator, with multiple lines and tubes in her swollen body. She had a probe protruding from her skull. This probe measured the pressure in her brain, and displayed it on a monitor above her bed. We would adjust her medications based on the pressure readings, with the goal of keeping the pressure down. If the pressure in her brain became too high, she risked permanent brain damage. As the brain swells inside the skull, the pressure increases due to the hard bone of the skull. It is not forgiving. It doesn't bend or adjust to accommodate…it just doesn't.

Over the next three days, the ICU doctors did all they could to try to save Ursela's life. Every day we had a "Wake up" period where the ventilator support was briefly stopped. We watched, in the hopes Ursela would begin to breathe on her own. We looked for any sign, no matter how small, that she was beginning to wake up. But the signs never came. Her family made the excruciating, yet extraordinarily generous decision to donate her organs.

This is where the work really began. Ursela was the first patient I had ever prepped for organ donation. The staff from the organ donor network showed up to assist in this process. They had a set of orders, and we had to follow them to the letter. When you are preparing a person to become an organ donor, you want the organs in the best shape possible. You want the blood pressure tightly controlled. You want the electrolytes (the sodium, potassium, the glucose) in normal range. We would draw labs, adjust fluids based on the results, and draw labs again the next hour.

While all this was occurring, the nurse from the donor network was frequently on the phone. Was there someone locally who needed a heart? Were they a good match with Ursela? If not, the calls would go to a wider and wider geographical area. We could hear the helicopter as it landed on the hospital roof, bringing a surgical organ retrieval team (the organ harvesting team). One call she made was to the eye bank.

When the gentleman from the eye bank arrived, he was very patient, and was kind enough to answer all my questions. I learned the eyes could be taken, and the corneas donated. This would be a blessed gift to someone who had lost their sight. The eyes could also be donated for research. He would take each eye – the entire eyeball – and place it in a container of saline (lightly salted water). Once done, he would take them back to the eye bank. The whole process would take less than an hour. "Ooh! Can I help?" I asked. Yes. He let me help.

Honestly, I didn't know if I would faint, if I would puke, but what the heck? It would be a once in a lifetime experience. I stood at the head of the bed as the gentleman explained the procedure. I was bravely holding the cup of saline. He had a clamp he placed inside the upper and lower eyelids, to keep them open. He had a set of knives with him. Then, he explained he would insert one of the knives at different points around the eyeball; he would aim the knife away from the eye, so as not to knick the eyeball itself. What he was doing was cutting each of the ocular muscles, so he could then remove the eyeball and place it in the cup. I had the all important job of screwing the lid on the cup.

At the time, I thought I was simply experiencing something "Way cool". As time went on, I realized it was a precious moment. This was another moment in Ursela's life when she gave of herself to help others, even in death. I feel honored to this day to have been a part of it.

$\mathscr{V}$ IS FOR VOMIT. $\mathscr{V}$ IS FOR VENEREAL
DISEASE, VENTILATOR, VERTIGO,
AND VAGINA.

$\mathscr{V}$ IS ALSO FOR VICTORIA.

Victoria was a 21-year-old female who came to our surgical depart-ment to have her gallbladder taken out. She had delivered a baby six weeks previously. Victoria was not the first postpartum female that I had seen for gallbladder issues. It is thought changes in hormones during pregnancy can cause the gallbladder to become sluggish, and lead to the formation of gallstones. This in turn can cause pain after eating, and nausea. The symptoms can become bothersome enough that the pesky organ needs to be removed.

When patients came in for surgery, we had a checklist we fol-lowed to get them ready. We had them sign a consent for the proce-dure. No consent, no surgery. We started an IV, placing a small needle in a vein and connecting it to a bag of fluid. Many people run around dehydrated at their baseline. Having them stop eating and drinking twelve hours before surgery can exacerbate this. We would run the fluids while waiting to send them off to the OR. The IV also served as an access for medications the patients would receive to start the anesthesia process, or to manage their pain. Patients received edu-cation on what to expect after surgery (trying to educate a sedated, painful patient doesn't work). There were three things we looked for that let us know patients were able to return home: they had to get out of bed and walk (with our help, of course), they had to be able to keep down fluids and small amounts of food – and by food I mean crackers and jelly – and they had to be able to urinate. Sometimes the bladder was the last part of the body to wake up and cooperate. A couple of patients a week would spend several hours with us because they couldn't pee.

As I was explaining these things to Victoria and her husband, she would say "Crackers? Forget that sh*t. I'm getting me some KFC when I wake up," to which I would reply, "I wouldn't recommend that. Not today."

The OR staff came to take Victoria to surgery. Her husband was allowed to follow her, only to a certain point. In order to maintain the cleanliness and sterility of the OR environment, he had to have a seat in the waiting room. Once they said their "See you laters", Victoria was wheeled through the surgical suite doors, and turned over to the operating room team.

I received a report from the recovery room staff. Victoria was doing well. She was awake, pain was under good control – and she was hungry. They had given her some crackers, but she told them she wanted to eat when she came back to the ambulatory surgery unit. Sure. I'll let her eat. Toast, crackers, jelly, fizzy pop. That was about all we kept in our department. If you wanted something significant to eat, patients were advised to wait until the next day and let the anesthesia work its way out of their systems to avoid issues with vomiting. Who wants to throw up after having any kind of abdominal surgery??

The nursing assistant and I checked Victoria over and got her settled in her room. We put some crackers and fizzy pop on her bedside table. We let her know we would be back to check on her, and I sat down to start putting together her discharge instructions. As the papers were being completed, I saw Victoria's husband coming down the hall, KFC in hand. I caught him before he went into her room and again reminded him she should not eat something so greasy and rich at this time. She should go easy, and she could have the KFC tomorrow. "Yeah," he said, "but my girl is hungry." Oh boy. OK.

It was time to recheck Victoria's vital signs, so I entered her room. Here she sat, a two-piece meal with mashed potatoes and gravy, cole slaw, nearly all gone. "How are you feeling?" I asked. "Good," she said. "I'm good." Vitals were normal. Telling her I would return in another fifteen minutes, I walked back to my desk, gently pulling her door closed behind me.

Did I mention V is for Vomit?

My buttcheeks were about an inch from my seat when I heard this loud sound. The door to her room came flying open and her boyfriend was wide eyed. "Ma'am, she's throwing up in there. She's throwing up bad." Now…. I'm not one to say I told you so, but the urge was there. The force was strong. I had to fight the force! I grabbed an emesis bag on my way to her room. We kept them in the rooms, but I wasn't sure what I was going to be facing. I wanted an extra, just in case. Poor Victoria was, in fact, throwing up. Chicken, potatoes, slaw. The smell was incredible. With one hand she was holding her abdomen, and with the other she was holding her emesis bag. She was moaning and sweaty. She didn't look so good anymore. I took her bag, gave her my empty one, and left to dispose of her bodily fluids using a HAZMAT approved method.

When I returned to her room, she was leaning back on her pillow, still breathing slightly heavy, saying, "Oh, man. Ooohhhh, man." This time when I asked how she was doing, I heard, "I probably shouldn't have done that. That was nasty".

Yes, Victoria . There is a smarty nurse. And she tried to tell you.

$\mathcal{W}$ IS FOR WOUND. $\mathcal{W}$ IS FOR WRIST,
WHITE MATTER, WOLFF-PARKINSON-WHITE
SYNDROME, AND WAIST.

$\mathcal{W}$ IS ALSO FOR WALTER.

Walter was an 83-year – old gentleman I met on my weekend rota-tion. He had been admitted the day before from our local state prison. Any of the prisoners needing medical attention came to our university hospital. The guards at the prison who knew Walter thought he was not acting like his usual self. He was a bit wobbly, and not as talkative as usual. He was brought to our ER, where he had labs and a head CT scan performed. The labs showed Walter was dehydrated, so IV fluids were started. The head CT did not show anything abnormal.

One unique challenge to his care was that Walter was hand-cuffed to his hospital bed. Both feet cuffed in order to prevent him from running away. The prisoners always were cuffed like this. I never knew what their crimes entailed and I didn't want to know. I didn't want it to influence my interactions with them. Whatever they had done, they had been through the court system and were now doing their time. My job was to attend to their medical needs. Whatever their crimes, they were people who had feelings, had families/ friends, and experienced pain. Who knows how they were treated in prison? The least I could do was treat them like human beings.

Every prisoner also had a guard with them. Depending on the patient, the guard might sit out in the hall just peering into the room at times. There were times, however, the guard was sitting right next to the patient's bed. This was so they could intervene quickly should the prisoner get out of hand. On one occasion while caring for a prisoner, I acknowledged the guard, then pulled the curtain so the patient could be examined in privacy. The next thing I knew, the curtain was being pulled back by the guard. Not knowing why the guard did that, I pulled the curtain again. Again the guard pulled the curtain, but this time he told me he needed to be able to see the prisoner at all times. Oh. OK. That made me a bit nervous....but, OK.

Walter was one of those prisoners whose guard could sit in the hallway. I mean, come on. Walter was 83. What on earth could he possibly do? He was friendly and quiet, not one of those patients who was on the call light every half hour.

I examined Walter at the start of my shift. Things appeared to be normal. As the day went on, he became sleepy and less responsive. His blood sugar was normal. I called the doctor and was given orders to get a STAT CT scan of the head. I had to push Walter in his bed over to the radiology department, which was on the opposite end of the hospital. We didn't have much staff on the unit that day, so the guard assisted me. As I was gathering what I needed to get Walter to CT scan, I asked the guard to uncuff Walter.

We were going to need to move him from the bed to the exam table. The guard told me he was not allowed to do that. He could only uncuff prisoners for urgent needs, so he would uncuff him once we got to the CT room. Seriously? My patient could be having a stroke at 83, and we still had to keep him cuffed?

As it turned out, Walter was indeed having a stroke. When patients present with stroke symptoms, oftentimes the initial scans don't show anything. If we repeat the scan in a few days, we may be able to pick up where a clot in the brain had settled, or where a vessel had burst and was bleeding. Walter had a clot in his brain. The radiologist pointed out to me where he saw some tissue that was actually dying. Walter's family was called, and they decided to make him a DNR, put him on comfort care, and let him go. AND…all the while he was dying, Walter continued to be cuffed to his bed. In my opinion, that is just unbelievable.

Walter did not pass away on my shift. I learned he died the next day. When I returned the next weekend for my Saturday shift, one of the nurses who was working the day he passed asked me if I knew why he was in prison. I started to tell her no, and I didn't want to know, when she blurted out, "He shot the man who raped his daughter".

You've got to be kidding me? Walter suffered emotionally knowing his daughter had been raped. Whether you believe he should have been in jail or not, I'm sure his days in prison were not all sunshine and lollipops. And his last days on this earth, unresponsive and dying, he was STILL in ankle cuffs. To this day, my heart gets heavy when I think of Walter that way.

# $\mathcal{X}$ IS FOR X-RAY. $\mathcal{X}$ IS FOR XANTHOMA, XIPHOID, X-CHROMOSOME, AND XANTHINE.

# $\mathcal{X}$ IS ALSO FOR XAVIER.

Xavier was a 21-year-old male who ended up in our rehab unit. Most of the patients we had were in an in-between stage – too healthy to be in the acute hospital, but too ill to be sent home. We would have patients who needed daily dressing changes on wounds but had no help at home. Due to insurance reasons – or the lack of – they did not qualify for home nursing, so they stayed with us. We had patients who needed chemo Monday through Friday, but lived one hundred miles away from our hospital. There was no way they could make a daily round trip drive like that, so…they stayed with us.

Xavier came to our unit after he had been in a high speed car accident. He had been running from the police when he lost control of a stolen car, and crashed. As a result of the crash, he broke his left lower leg and right ankle. Both were in casts, rendering him wheel-chair bound. He would be on our unit for at least six weeks getting physical therapy, and being frequently monitored by the orthopedic team. Once he was healed enough and cleared by orthopedics, Xavier's next stop was jail.

At the time he was in our unit, patients had the ability to sign off the unit and walk around the hospital, even go outside. In his case, Xavier would get in a wheelchair and push himself outside. On the weekends, patients who were in the inpatient drug/alcohol rehab unit would come to our unit. I suppose it was a way of saving money?

The hospital could close a unit and not have to pay for staffing three shifts. Rumors were that the drug/alcohol patients would go outside and find, hidden in bushes, drugs/alcohol their friends left for them. So much for rehab (although I was not able to verify this myself). I was working weekends. One Saturday when I returned to work, a fellow nurse had a disturbing story for me. One of our patients had signed himself out on a weeknight. Apparently he walked a few blocks to a convenience store and bought himself some alcohol. How much, I don't know. It was enough, however, for him to be found floating face down in our river. Luckily, he lived.

During one particularly busy weekend shift, we were full of patients needing lots of attention – wound dressings needed to be changed, IV antibiotics needed to be hung, trachs needed to be cleaned, and patients kept coming up to the nurses' station for various reasons. Some just wanted water, others wanted their pain meds (remember rehab?). We were a twenty eight bed unit. We typically had one RN and one nursing assistant for fourteen patients. At times, we also had a floating nurse who helped on the unit wherever it was needed. We would attempt to check on each patient every two hours, just poking our heads into the rooms to see if they needed anything – and were still breathing. This particular shift, I assessed Xavier in the morning. It was almost noon before I could get a chance to get back to his room.

When I got there, it looked like someone had tried to rob him. The sheets on the bed were disheveled, his hospital gown was on the bed, and cards he had received from friends and his girlfriend were out of their envelopes, hastily tossed aside. I asked other staff and even the ambulatory patients if they had seen him. No one could recall seeing him since that morning. Great! We checked the sign out log. Xavier had indeed signed himself out – four hours earlier. Because he had not returned, we went back to his room and started looking for anything that might tell us where he might be. We found it. In reading some of the cards he had received from his girlfriend, we discovered she had been sending him money. Just a few dollars with each card, so as not to draw suspicion – but enough for him to get a bus ticket, hop a bus, and get out of town. HE. WAS. GONE. Apparently, Xavier thought sneaking his way out of town would keep him from going to jail.

I had to notify the nursing supervisor to tell her we "lost" a patient. That's always a pleasant thing to have to do. NOT! In turn, she notified the police. Within a few hours, a couple of uniformed officers came to our unit and were combing through Xavier's room themselves. They did not share any information with us. I assume they were able to gather information that would lead them to Xavier's trail?

Needless to say, after this episode, privileges to leave the unit were suspended, leading to a whole host of unhappy patients. Shortly after, I left that particular unit and found another position in order to go back to school. I had heard the unit was totally closed and the patients redistributed among the many other units in the hospital – none having sign out sheets.

# $\mathscr{Y}$ IS FOR YELLOW FEVER. $\mathscr{Y}$ IS FOR Y CHROMOSOME, YEAST, YOLK SAC, AND YAWNING.

# $\mathscr{Y}$ IS ALSO FOR YERSENIA.

Yersenia was a 43-year-old Spanish speaking patient who came to see me in our busy clinic. I had only been a practitioner for eight months when she showed up in one of my exam rooms. With the help of the interpreter, I conducted my usual questioning – what are the symptoms, when did they start, how long have they been going on?

My medical assistant told me Yersenia was here with complaints of dizziness. Being new, I poured as fast as I could through all the resources I had: what causes dizziness, what tests should I order, what can I do for her in the five minutes I had her here in the clinic?

Our clinic was an FQHC – a Federally Qualified Healthcare Center. We were obligated to provide care to anyone who wanted to be seen in our clinic. We had people with insurance, people without. We had single people, single parents, married couples, gay, straight. We also had many immigrants in the community coming to the clinic. I saw patients from Mexico, Africa, Korea, and Vietnam. I always enjoyed the visits as I took them as an opportunity to learn one new thing. Some of the things I learned – I wish I could unlearn.

Back to Yersenia. She was answering my questions. She has been feeling weak and dizzy for the past twenty four hours. She told me she typically drank six eight ounce cups of water a day. The room was not spinning. She was not on any blood pressure medications.

She didn't have any ear pain or sinus issues. She didn't have any urinary tract symptoms. As I was going through my list of questions, I heard this quiet voice from the corner of the room say, "She's dizzy because she hasn't eaten in three days." It was the interpreter. "I'm sorry – say that again." She told me again, "Yersenia is dizzy because she hasn't had anything to eat in three days." "Yersenia," I said surprisedly, "why haven't you eaten in three days?" She gave her answer in Spanish, and the interpreter told me, "They were running out of food, and she wanted her children to be able to eat, so she gave them the food."

Now, this wasn't 1920. She wasn't a single woman who lost her husband and now had to figure out how to feed her family. This was 2016 for heaven's sake. 2016, and we still had people who couldn't provide enough food for their family. How disgraceful.

I don't know your thoughts, but this is not a female, immigrant-who-stole-my-job, they deserve it kinda thing. This is a human thing. This is a humanitarian issue. How can we continue to have people in society, any society, who cannot even have enough food to eat?! We have restaurants who serve $50 steaks, and children go hungry? We have grocery stores throwing out produce that isn't "pretty" anymore, and people are going days without eating?

I have to say the staff in my clinic were top notch. They were kind, caring people who were there because they loved people and wanted to help them.

When they heard of Yersenia's situation, the staff pulled together. Some made food to take to her home. Some donated money and grocery gift cards. Their actions warmed my heart. I was able to get a social worker involved, who gave Yersenia a list of local agencies who were also able to provide assistance, so something like this would not have to happen again.

But she is just one patient. How many more patients, people out there going through the same thing? If you can only do one good thing today, donate to a food bank. Donate a grocery store gift card to a homeless shelter. Check out the Too Good to Go app and help end food waste. Buy some nonperishable foods and donate to a local grade school so children in your community don't have to go hungry.

One job loss, one missed paycheck, and it could be you. It could.

*Z* IS FOR ZINC. *Z* IS FOR ZENKER DIVERTICULUM, ZIKA VIRUS, ZOLLINGER-ELLISON SYNDROME, AND ZYGOTE.

*Z* IS ALSO FOR ZENYA.

Zenya was a 76-year-old female who had moved to the US from her native country six years before we met. She had come here after her husband died to live with her daughter and son-in-law.

I met Zenya in the endoscopy suite at our community hospital. She was in our unit that day to have a colon decompression. What fun!

In her native country, Zenya's diet was healthy. She ate fresh fruits and vegetables every day. She cooked her own food at home. She was active and walked to a farmers market several days a week. Once moving in with her daughter, things changed. Her daughter was afraid she would fall, so she told Zenya she didn't want her outside walking alone. This presented a challenge as her daughter worked during the day, leaving Zenya limited to the confines of the house, and the yard. Thinking she was doing her mother a favor, she told Zenya she didn't have to do the cooking. She wanted Zenya to relax, so many nights her daughter would pick up fast food on the way home from work. Some nights, they went out to eat.

As a result of these changes to her routine over time, Zenya's health started to change. Since coming to the US she had put on thirty pounds. Her doctor had wanted her to take a statin for her elevated LDL, but she declined. Her bowels started slowing down, and now a part of her daily routine was taking stool softeners and stimulants – things she had never even heard of in her country. For the most part, Zenyawas compliant with these. Some days, her daughter told us, she just thought it was stupid so she would not take the bowel meds. And here she was, in our endo unit.

Zenya was starting to feel bloated and distended, so her daughter had her take some powdered laxative. When it didn't work, her daughter had her take a magnesium laxative. It helped just a tiny bit. When she still complained of abdominal discomfort a few days later, Zenya's daughter brought her to the ER. An X Ray was done which showed her to be very constipated. The exact wording on the X Ray report was "very large stool burden".

One of our GI doctors (GI tract specialists) was consulted. He determined it was best to take Zenya to the GI lab, and perform a colon decompression. Colon decompression is done when a patient's colon is blocked, and stool is not passing. If the stool load becomes too large, there can be dangerous consequences such as perforated bowel (a hole in the wall of the colon, which leads to waste leaking into the abdomen).

A colon decompression is done similar to colonoscopy – except in this case, there is stool in the colon the physician has to try to maneuver a scope around. The colon is not empty and clean. The patient is sedated and the physician slowly advances his scope to the point where the large and small intestine meet.

At this point in the procedure, a long thin tube is passed through the scope. We can instill water through the tube, to try to stimulate the colon to evacuate. We can also instill medication such as powdered laxative or magnesium containing laxative. At times, we can encounter some elevated pressure in the colon, which causes air and liquid stool to come out the end of the tube. The physician slowly pulls back on his scope as his assistant feeds the decompression tube, just as slowly, forward to prevent it from being pulled out of the patient. This particular day, I was the "tube feeder".

I had only done this procedure one other time, with another physician. The physician I was working with during Zenya's procedure was not known for having a sense of humor. As we were maneuvering our respective tubes, he said,"You'd better stand back." I chuckled a little, thinking he was trying to make a funny. He wasn't. All he said was, "I'm serious." As if in slow motion, just as I stepped to the side, from the tube came this high powered squirt of brown, highly odorous fluid. Whew! Dodged that one – sort of. We had the lights dimmed during the procedure so we could see our monitor more clearly. Once the procedure was done, we turned up the lights and got Zenya ready to go to the recovery room.

Behind us in each room was a set of cabinets where we kept our supplies. My best guess is the cabinets were located six feet behind us. As I turned to set the scope on our procedure cart, I couldn't believe what I saw. Dripping down the front of the cabinets was brown liquid – the brown liquid that shot out of Zenya. I was extremely grateful the doctor told me to stand back. If I hadn't moved, it would have been all over me. What I wasn't so grateful for was the next hour I spent opening every drawer in those cabinets, cleaning up Zenya's poop.

I'm hoping after this procedure she was more faithful about taking her stool meds.